Fitness Equipment for Beginners

How and When to use gym equipment

By PROSENCE

ABOUT PROSENCE

Our Mission

We are dedicated to guiding, motivating and providing the tools necessary to transform people into the best version of themselves. Our goal is to empower men and women across the globe to realize that physical and mental fitness are not a short-term solution, but a lifetime choice, and to actualize what they have come to understand into a daily routine. We invite you to discover this process for yourself as you join us in the exploration of science-based knowledge that can lead to better health, greater fulfillment and astonishing vitality.

Who is Prosence?

Hi, I'm Antonio Mazzotta - certified Fitness Trainer and health enthusiast, and the founder of Prosence. While I don't think I'll ever turn down mom's homemade pasta and pizza, as an Italian living in Switzerland I've built a life dedicated to health and fitness. Now, I want to share the secrets to my success with you.

I got involved in this industry over 7 years ago, and quickly developed a passion for all things health and fitness. I knew right away that this is what I was born to do and haven't looked back. My days are spent developing new routines, training hard and meeting other fitness-minded and health-conscious individuals. I love working with my clients and coaching about weight training, dieting and healthy lifestyle choices. My number one priority is motivating people to achieve any fitness goal they seek. Whether you're looking to lose weight, get stronger, build cardio and endurance or just maintain overall health and vitality - I'm here to get you to your goals.

My team and I work hard to dispel the health and fitness myths and misinformation clogging the Internet today. We're driven by the desire to offer you a safe and manageable yet powerfully effective path to the best health of your life. Prosence is firmly committed to motivating, inspiring, and educating through the sharing of objective, fact-based health and fitness information that is rooted in science. We give you the tools you need to get in great shape and build a lifetime of good health.

Join us - let's work together to maximize your potential and achieve your optimal self while embracing life to the fullest!

Learn more on our website: www.prosencefitness.com, blog and keep up with the daily education and motivation by liking us on Twitter, Facebook & Instagram @prosencefitness.

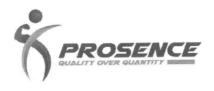

Table of Contents

Introduction

Embarking on a fitness journey can be pretty intimidating. There are so many new things to learn and even a slight misapplication can make it harder for an exerciser to reach their goals. Of all the choices a new exerciser faces in their training, equipment selection can be the most daunting. Does it really make a difference if you perform a bench press with a barbell or dumbbell? If so, what's the difference? Should my training consist of mostly resistance bands? What about mostly resistance machines? These questions come up all the time in the minds of beginners. But don't worry, we here at Prosence will be here to guide you.

Let's get started.

Chapter 1

Importance of Variety In Exercise

It is important to tailor training towards a specific goal when exercising, but that doesn't mean variety can't be beneficial. Variety in exercise selection usually refers to the inclusion of multiple different movement patterns targeting different muscles. But it can also refer to the alteration of movement patterns or loading by changing the implement/equipment used. By using different implements it becomes possible for the same movement pattern to provide an entirely different effect to the body. This can be seen when comparing a barbell bench press to a dumbbell bench press. The dumbbell variation allows for there to be greater range of motion, allowing the pectorals to stretch more at the bottom of the rep and also cause each rep to last slightly longer.

Additionally, it is possible for some movement patterns to only be performed with certain implements and not with others. This can be easily demonstrated by considering the pullup. The pullup can be performed with a pullup bar, but it is impossible to use a dumbbell alone to do a pullup. Having access to multiple implements allows an exerciser to have more freedom in designing/choosing their workout routine.

In general, having a routine that uses 1-4 types of implements is typically ideal (though this range is flexible and some good routines can have more than 4). It isn't absolutely necessary for a good routine to use more than one implement, but strategically incorporating multiple when appropriate can improve the effects of a workout routine. Having too many types of implements in a routine can be counterproductive in that it can slow strength gains.

Chapter 2

Barbell

The barbell is by far the most common and useful piece of equipment in any gym. It is highly versatile, facilitates the use of a lot of weight, is available in almost every gym, and is the most long term cost effective piece of equipment for a home gym.

But what is a barbell? A barbell is a straight long iron bar. Barbells typically come in one of two forms. They can either be designed with a fixed load or with a variable load. Fixed load barbells typically have large cylindrical weights attached to either side that cannot be removed. A label can usually be found somewhere on the bar indicating its weight (e.g. 40 lbs, 50 lbs, etc.). Variable load barbells typically weigh 45 pounds and have areas on either end where weight plates can be attached to determine the absolute load used during a movement. They often come with clips that can be used to prevent the weight plates from sliding off during an exercise, increasing safety.

Variable load barbells are by far superior to fixed load barbells given their resistance can be acutely manipulated and they don't often provide an upper limit. Most gyms do not have infinite resources such as space or money, so they invest in a small number of fixed load barbells limiting the loading options of those using them. It is common for gyms to only have loads up to a certain weight (e.g. 100 lbs), and to have larger increments between loads available with heavier barbells (e.g. having 90 lb and 100 lb barbells, but no 95 lb barbells).

Variable load barbells on the other hand can typically be adjusted in 5 lb increments (by adding 2.5 lb plates to both sides of the bar) to a maximum capacity of 400+ lbs with weight limits varying depending on the specific variable load barbell used. They provide much more freedom and allow for greater progression within and control of exercise programs. Given weight plates are placed on either side to select the load used during an exercise, it is also the most affordable long term option for home gym goers. By purchasing two 2.5 lb plates, two 5 lb plates, four 10 lb plates, two 25 lb plates, and three 45 pound plates, a variable loading barbell can be adjusted to any 5 lb increment between 45 lbs and 420 lbs. This can allow for a lifetime of lifting and progression. The latter is important given adaptation to exercise stress only comes with a progression in the difficulty of exercise (this is typically done through increasing the load/weight used). It is hard to consistently increase weight on a fixed load barbell because the load is fixed and increasing means purchasing a new slightly heavier barbell every time an exerciser gets slightly stronger.

From here on out in the section, the term barbell will refer exclusively to variable load barbells unless otherwise specified. They are by far more common, more practical, and more standardized. The use of a barbell typically involves both limbs working simultaneously on moving/manipulating the same object. Because force can be produced through multiple limbs and act on the same object, exercisers tend to lift larger loads with the barbell than most other implements. If an exerciser can perform a movement with 100 pounds in each hand, they can typically lift well over 200 lbs in the barbell version of that movement. Lifting larger loads means that there is a greater overall stress on systems of the body such as the endocrine, vascular, and musculoskeletal systems. Stimulating bone growth typically requires a significant amount of weight, which is most easily achieved through the use of a barbell. Furthermore, the large loads lifted in barbell movements lead to greater hormonal responses to training (e.g. leading to more muscle building) and return more blood to the heart from the rest of the body.

Because barbell exercises allow for the use of significant weight and are often the most productive pieces of a workout, they should usually be placed towards the beginning of a workout day. If done at the very end, fatigue from other less productive movements can limit performance. It should be noted that multi-joint barbell movements that allow an exerciser to lift very heavy weight should be done early on such as the high bar barbell back squat, the barbell conventional deadlift, or the barbell bench press. Single joint barbell movements like the barbell biceps curl, the barbell skull crusher, or the barbell shrug should be performed towards the end of a workout.

Chapter 3

Dumbbell

Dumbbells are typically considered the second most common implement and can be seen as mini barbells. They are small free weights that allow for a ton of variety and can mimic almost all of the movements an exerciser can do when using a barbell. As an example, an exerciser can do a barbell bench press or a dumbbell bench press. They can do a barbell overhead press or a dumbbell overhead press. They can do a barbell bent over row or a dumbbell bent over row. It is advantageous that they are similar because it allows weakness in specific movement patterns with one implement to be addressed by using the other.

But what is a dumbbell? A dumbbell can come in one of two forms similar to a barbell. It can be designed with a fixed load or variable load, though fixed load dumbbells are actually more common. Aside from that, they are like miniature one-handed barbells. The only important differences are that they hold lower absolute loads because less force is applied to each individual implement, they allow for limbs to move independently of each other, and they allow for greater range of motion during some movements.

The use of dumbbells can benefit muscular imbalances given they train one limb at a time. If a muscle on one side of the body had grown excessively weak due to an injury or imbalance in past training, more sets can be performed with the weaker limb to balance strength between both sides. Correcting imbalances can prevent future injuries. In training one limb at a time, there is also typically greater involvement of abdominal musculature given they have to work to stabilize the movement. It is uncommon and difficult to perform one limbed movements with a barbell, so dumbbells are typically required to train in this way and facilitate ab development/strength.

Because dumbbells allow for greater range of motion during some movements, they can allow for reps to last longer, increasing the time a muscle spends under tension. As time under tension increases, muscular hypertrophy usually increases.

Given dumbbell movements don't allow for the use of as much weight as their barbell counterparts, they are typically placed in the middle of a workout. Of course, single-joint movements should still be grouped towards the end of a workout.

Chapter 4

Kettlebell

Kettlebells are most commonly used in metabolic conditioning style workouts. They can be held with either one or two hands and their design allows for some but not all barbell and dumbbell movements to be mimicked.

But what is a kettlebell? A kettlebell is a weighted iron ball connected to a curved handle. The implement is typically small and all kettlebell weights are fixed. Heavier kettlebells tend to have larger balls and larger handles for gripping. The position of the iron ball allows for unique movements like kettlebell swings to be performed. By far kettlebell swings are the most advantageous kettlebell exercise and one of the only movements that is justified to be performed with a kettlebell over another implement.

Kettlebell swings use similar hip, knee, and trunk muscles to the barbell and dumbbell deadlifts. They can be used as excellent ways to bring up deadlift strength, and they even carry over to squat strength. Though in terms of muscular development, kettlebell swings are phenomenal at glute development. Given a majority of the force produced to drive kettlebells upwards comes from the glutes, swings can play a pivotal role in building a large butt.

Though kettlebell swings are the most prominent and heavily researched kettlebell movement, kettlebells can also be used as replacements for certain dumbbell movements when a dumbbell is not available. They can replace movements like dumbbell goblet squats, dumbbell overhead squats, dumbbell romanian deadlifts, and more.

Chapter 5

Resistance Bands/Cables

Resistance bands and cables are two distinct forms of resistance but can both provide for needed accessory movements in a routine. Resistance bands are considered variable resistance training and cables are considered machine based resistance training (though in some cases, cable pulley systems are designed to be variable).

But what are they? Resistance bands are stretchy rubber/elastic bands that provide resistance to a movement by either attaching to another implement or an exerciser's limbs directly. They provide variable resistance in that they provide more resistance the more they are stretched. This leads to less of a training stimulus at the beginning of the range of motion and more of one towards the end. Typically, this isn't conducive to success given the training stimulus for the lower part of the range of motion is often insignificant. Cables however are pulley systems attached to weight stacks. There is typically either a specific or changeable handle at the end of a cable to allow an exerciser to customize their exercise. When using a cable, resistance can be selected by changing the position of a pin on the weight stack it is attached to. Cables may or may not have variable resistance given some machines are designed to decrease machine resistance during certain parts of the range of motion and others are not. Because of this, a weight that is manageable for a movement on one cable machine may not be manageable on another.

Cables typically come in multiple designs to allow for different movements to be performed. Some are overhead and positioned above a seat to allow for movements like the wide grip lat pulldown or reverse close grip lat pulldown. Others are positioned in line with a bench to allow for cable seated rows, and others can have their handle position adjusted to any height along a vertical column. Depending on the movement one would like to perform they would have to seek out the matching cable system. Given each comes with its own weight stack, there are usually a variety of loads that can be selected on each cable machine allowing for adequate progression as an exerciser gets stronger. In terms of exercise selection cables can mimic some movements that can be performed with barbell or dumbbell implements but not all. Furthermore they allow for unique movements to be performed like the tricep rope pushdown, hip abduction, or hip adduction.

Bands have fixed tensile strength meaning that the range of resistance they can be provided as they are stretched out is fixed and based on the band itself. When compared to more traditional training methods bands often don't provide similar gains in strength or muscle mass. This can be largely attributed to the lower absolute loads that are used during the parts of the range of motion before the band is more stretched. However, when resistance bands are used to replace at least a fifth of a regular training load on a barbell, it can lead to increases in power output. Power can be defined as the rate of force development. The higher an exerciser's power output is, the faster they produce force. It isn't the same as strength because strength is independent of time and relates to the total amount of force produced.

In workout design, cable movements should typically be placed closer to the end of a workout, grouping multi joint movements earlier on and single joint movements later on. Resistance band movements should typically not be included in a workout at all, but if they are included for the sake of power development they should be added to the first large multi joint barbell movement.

Furthermore, in terms of cost effectiveness for home gym goers, neither cables nor resistance bands are worth the cost if resources are limited. Cables allow for some additional movements to be performed but take up alot of space and can require multiple types of cables to perform all cable movements. Bands are fixed resistance training devices and multiple need to be bought for the sake of progression. Though even if multiple bands are bought, their positive effects will likely be minimal at best.

Chapter 6

TRX

The TRX has become one of the most popular modern fads. It's hip, it's cool, and it's iconically colored. It is a versatile training system that most gym goers can recognize but few know how to actually use.

But what is a TRX and how does it work? A TRX is a suspension system that allows for modified bodyweight movements to be performed given the only resistance is bodyweight. When using the TRX, the angle at which the body is to the ground typically determines the resistance for most movements. The less steep the angle, the more difficult/highly loaded a movement will be. For example, if performing a TRX pushup with feet on the ground, the movement will be harder closest to parallel to the ground. The same would be true of performing an inverted bodyweight TRX row.

TRX implements can be seen as an add-on to bodyweight training. They allow for resistance of bodyweight movements to be altered in a way that can reduce their loading. This can be an invaluable training tool for those that struggle with bodyweight versions of a movement. If performing a bodyweight pushup is too difficult, a TRX assisted pushup may be manageable until the exerciser progresses to a regular pushup. Similarly performing a single leg TRX squat can be used as a stepping stone to a regular single leg squat. The movements that are unique to the TRX and bodyweight movements made more difficult by the TRX, usually involve abdominal training.

The one big issue with the TRX is that given its loading parameters it isn't helpful for stimulating bone growth. As most people age, their bone density decreases. This can lead to severe limitations later on in life and large decreases are especially prevalent in women. Because TRX training doesn't promote very much bone growth, it is recommended that it be performed alongside more traditional resistance training methods like barbell or dumbbell use. If used in a routine, it should be placed towards the middle or end, before single joint movements.

Chapter 7

Sandbags

Sandbags are uncommon implements that are most often seen used by military and law enforcement groups. Given their unorthodox nature they tend to create instability during movement patterns that leads to a unique stimulus.

But what are sandbags? They are bags filled with sand or some other rough material to increase the weight of the bag. Sandbags are relatively short but dense and often bend/twist based on the way they are held, giving them a non-fixed form.

Sandbags allow for resistance to be added to a movement in a way that increases the activation of stabilizer muscles given it often loads the body in unique and uneven ways. This can lead to greater abdominal/trunk development and increase the endurance of those muscles. This is especially important for soldiers and law enforcement who prepare to perform long-duration physical activity under uncertain conditions and need to operate efficiently. If they need to drag/carry another person or a large object for a long distance, sandbag training can help them. Aside from increasing the muscular endurance of stabilizers, it also acclimates an individual to getting used to carrying an awkward object. This is also one of the reasons it is sometimes found in the training programs of strongman competitors as it can help them prepare for many of the awkward movements they perform in competition.

Though there hasn't been a large amount of research conducted regarding sandbag training, it is still anecdotally and logically promising for those who plan to put themselves in tough unstable conditions. This can even include casual competitors of popular obstacle courses like ninja warrior.

Sandbag training can be a bit pricey to maintain in a home gym environment because a single hole in a bag can be enough reason to warrant a replacement. If any small amount of material leaks out before fixed then the loading of the bag will change. Given it is easy for bags to rupture it is reasonable to assume replacement sandbags will be needed at some point in an exerciser's training career.

Chapter 8

Bodyweight

Bodyweight training is extremely common because it can be done anywhere. Even exercisers that exclusively use barbells, dumbbells, and cables in their regular routines resort to bodyweight training when they go on vacation. More than anything else, it is convenient.

But what is bodyweight training? It is a form of training where the only resistance used is bodyweight. This is inclusive of movements where external equipment is used as long as no additional resistance is added (e.g. pullup bars, dip bars, and TRX). Typically though, the body is exclusively in contact with the floor, a box, or a bench during bodyweight movements. Bodyweight training allows for a moderate amount of variety, but it has several limitations when performed without access certain implements like a pullup bar or TRX.

Due to the nature of bodyweight training, resistance can't be selected in a way to allow for consistent progression in load given that bodyweight is the resistance and can't be significantly changed within an exercise session. Because of this, progression when performing bodyweight training of any type has to occur through modifications of an exercise's movement pattern. If an exerciser needs to increase resistance from that provided by a standard pushup, they can progress by raising one leg in the air and turning it into a more difficult movement. This form of progression has severe limitations given it doesn't allow for small consistent increases in load, and loading can only be increased by changing the movement pattern. There is only so much resistance that can be provided by bodyweight though because it is a finite value. This typically does not pose a problem for beginner or intermediate exercisers. But advanced and elite athletes may not be able to receive an adequate training stimulus from certain types of bodyweight movements.

Of additional concern is that certain muscles can't be targeted with just access to a floor or box when performing bodyweight movements. A large majority of muscles on the back and the elbow flexor muscle group cannot be targeted by bodyweight exercises without access to a TRX or a pullup bar. It is extremely important that all routines train the entire body in a balanced fashion. If only part of the body is trained, eventual muscle imbalances will develop. This can lead to injury, chronic pain, and other health issues long term. If the back and elbow flexors can't be trained through bodyweight alone, they should still be trained by using any other implement.

When being programmed into a resistance training routine, bodyweight movements can be placed at any point based on their difficulty and relative intensity. Bodyweight movements that can only be performed for a small number of reps (3-5) should be placed earlier on. Those that can be performed for a larger number of reps (10-15) should be placed toward the end of a workout.

Though it is important to note that bodyweight training involves cardio. If all an exerciser has is their bodyweight, they can walk, run, or sprint in dozens of different cardio programs. It is more difficult to perform cardio with external resistance than with bodyweight alone and thereby most common for cardio to be performed with just bodyweight.

Chapter 9

Frequently Asked Questions

Can I use a barbell with one hand?

It is possible to perform one handed exercises using a barbell. Though the neuromuscular coordination this requires, the minimum weight of a typical variable loaded barbell being 45 pounds, and the length of a typical barbell make one handed movements very difficult to perform properly. If performed, stabilizer muscles will be more active and a unique unstable stimulus will be provided.

If performing a single handed barbell movement like the barbell turkish get-up or the one arm barbell deadlift, it is important to place the hand at the exact center of the barbell. Being at the center of mass will prevent the bar from tilting laterally out of the hand and come crashing down.

Can I just increase the number of reps with a bodyweight movement to progress instead of modifying the movement pattern?

Unfortunately, this would not work. Given that the number of reps performed in a movement is inverse the intensity of the movement. When exercising, training should be at certain intensities to elicit certain adaptations. If an exercise can be performed for more reps, it means its intensity has decreased. This typically occurs when an exerciser gets stronger or the external load (bodyweight) decreases. In order to maintain the same type of stimulus, the movement should be of a greater intensity and performed for the same number of reps. As an example, when training in a low rep range (<6 reps), muscular strength tends to improve the most. When training in a high rep range (>12 reps), muscular endurance tends to improve the most. This is in part because the intensity of a movement determines which muscle fibers will be involved with the movement and the specific role they'll play during the movement. Though this is also related to the hormonal, or endocrine, response to training. Higher intensity training tends to lead to greater secretion of anabolic hormones like human growth hormone and testosterone. Greater concentrations of these facilitate muscle building and prevent muscle wasting. As reps increase and intensity decreases, these responses would eventually get minimized (e.g. they respond less to 20 reps than 8 reps). Though it is tricky to navigate, thousands of modifications for bodyweight movements can be found in databases online. These can be used to simplify the process of progression with bodyweight movements without having to increase reps and decrease intensity.

What do I do if I'm not strong enough to lift a variable load barbell without any additional weight plates on it?

This is a very common issue for exercisers who are just starting out. Fortunately, most exercisers can lift more than the weight of a 45 lb variable loaded barbell for a majority of their movements after the first month or two of training. If it is not possible to perform a movement with a barbell starting out, it is recommended that the movement be performed with a dumbbell instead. This should continue until the muscular strength developed from the dumbbell movement is enough to allow the easy use of a 45 lb variable loaded barbell. It is typically safe to move on to a regular barbell once at least 20 lb dumbbells are being used for the movement. Given the barbell and dumbbell can be used for very similar movement patterns there is a replacement for almost every barbell movement imaginable and there should not be an issue with substituting in an exact dumbbell replica of the movement.

Can I just use weight plates as implements on their own? They are a form of resistance.

It is possible to use a weight plate as an implement if needed, but it is usually not beneficial. Given their shape and size, they cannot be used with many movement patterns. If they can be used for a movement pattern, their loading is fixed which can lead to later issues with progression. Though not typical, it is most common for plates to be used during special types of forearm and grip training. They are used in grip training because plates tend to be thick and thicker objects are harder to hold on to. The harder the forearms and hands have to work to hold on to an object, the greater muscle activation and growth there tends to be.

It is also about as common to see weight plates used as resistance for sit ups and other movements similar to sit ups. Though it can increase resistance during a movement like the sit up, it is advised that this be done carefully. Many exercisers round their backs to hold their weight plate during the sit up and doing so is not ideal.

Conclusion

I hope that this overview of equipment will in some way serve to provide all of you out there with the foundation for future success. The largest barrier for many prospective exercisers out there is that it's really hard to stay motivated when they don't really know what they're doing. By helping you out here and providing valuable information about the tools available to you, our aim is that you will be able to have certainty in your training, and that it will help you stay on track.

Seeing as we've reached the end of our journey, it's important that you use the information you've learned here. With the confidence you'd built in the types of equipment available, go out and try different exercises with them! Do a dumbbell bench press. Then, a day later, do a barbell one! The best way to reinforce what you've learned and make sure you don't forget is to start working with the equipment. Once you work with them long enough, the differences between implements will be second nature to you.

Thank you for purchasing this book, I hope you enjoyed it.

Finally, if you enjoyed this book then I'd like to ask you for a favor. Will you be kind enough to leave a review for this book on Amazon? It would be greatly appreciated!

Don't forget to follow us on Twitter, Facebook & Instagram and visit our website www.prosencefitness.com to get empowered, educated and inspired to become the best version of yourself in life! You deserve it.

References

1. Haff, G., & Triplett, N. T. (2016). Essentials of strength training and conditioning. Champaign, IL: Human Kinetics.

2. Smith, F. (1982). Strength Training Modes: Dynamic Variable Resistance and the Universal System. National Strength Coaches Association Journal, 4(4), 14. doi:10.1519/0199-610x(1982)004<0014:dvratu>2.3.co;2

3. Farias, D. D., Willardson, J. M., Paz, G. A., Bezerra, E. D., & Miranda, H. (2017). Maximal Strength Performance and Muscle Activation for the Bench Press and Triceps Extension Exercises Adopting Dumbbell, Barbell, and Machine Modalities Over Multiple Sets. Journal of

Strength and Conditioning Research, 31(7), 1879-1887. doi:10.1519/jsc.0000000000001651

4. Garhammer, J. (1981). Strength Training Modes: Free Weight Equipment for the Development of Athletic strength and power—Part I. National Strength Coaches Association Journal, 3(6), 24. doi:10.1519/0199-610x(1981)003<0024:fweftd>2.3.co;2

5. Hughes, D. E., Cockerham, G., & Paul, J. S. (2006). Encouraging inclusive design through standardisation. Designing Accessible Technology, 21-30.

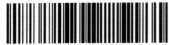

Printed in Great Britain
by Amazon